Bruno Grön

CW00402764

Heal your:
A Guide to Self-Healing

Chapter title:

Foreword

Welcome to "Heal Yourself: A Guide to Self-Healing" by Bruno Gröning. By picking up this book, you've already taken the first step on a remarkable journey – a journey that has the potential to change your life in many ways.

In a world dominated by technological advances and medical breakthroughs, we often forget the innate power of our own bodies and minds to heal ourselves. This book serves as a reminder and guide to harness this often neglected but incredibly powerful resource.

The chapters of this book are carefully designed to cover a wide range of topics relevant to self-healing. From the importance of a healthy diet and physical activity to the more subtle aspects such as stress management, positive relationships, and the power of self-love. Each chapter is a building block that helps you develop a comprehensive understanding of the various factors that affect your health and well-being.

The book emphasizes that health is not just the absence of disease, but a state of complete physical, mental and social well-being. It emphasizes the role of prevention and encourages you to be proactive, rather than just responding to health challenges as they arise.

Science has already confirmed what many cultures and traditions have known for centuries: our psyche and immune system are powerful allies on the path to healing. This book provides you with the tools to better understand and use these inner forces.

It is important to emphasize that this book is not intended as a substitute for professional medical advice or treatment. Rather, it is meant to be a supplement that helps you become an active participant in your own healing process.

No matter where you are in your health journey, this book offers practical advice and insights that will empower you to make more conscious choices for your health. It's never too early or too late to take control of your own well-being.

We hope that "Heal Yourself" will be not only an informative read for you, but also an inspiring experience. May it give you the courage and insight you need to unleash the remarkable power of self-healing in your own life.

Introduction: The power of self-healing

Self-healing is a fundamental part of the human experience. Although modern medicine has made incredible progress, our body's ability to heal itself remains one of its most powerful qualities. This book is a comprehensive guide to using and improving this skill.

The power of self-healing is a reality that has been confirmed by countless scientific studies. It can be seen in everyday experiences such as healing cuts and broken bones, but it can also be used for more serious health problems.

The key to promoting self-healing lies in our understanding of health and disease. Health is not just the absence of disease, but a state of complete physical, mental and social well-being. Disease is often the result of imbalances in one or more of these areas.

In this book, we will explore these areas in detail and present concrete strategies and techniques to promote your health and prevent or treat diseases. While we recognize the importance of medical care, the focus of this book is on preventive measures and supporting the body's natural healing processes.

We will not only cover physical aspects such as diet and exercise, but also mental and emotional components. We will highlight the importance of sleep and rest and explore the value of naturopathy and traditional healing methods.

In addition, we will explore the role of relationships and social life, as well as the importance of mindfulness and spirituality in health and well-being.

This guide is designed to be suitable for people of all ages and stages of life. It's never too early or too late to take control of your health and help your body heal.

Remember that each body is unique, and therefore there is no "one-size-fits-all". It is important that you learn to listen to your body and adapt the advice and techniques in this book to your individual needs and circumstances.

Health is a journey, not a destination. It's an ongoing process that requires dedication, patience, and often experimentation. Be kind to yourself and remember that every small improvement can make a big difference.

Chapter 2: Body Awareness: Understanding Your Own Physiology

Our body is a complex system of interconnected organs and processes. To cure it effectively, we need to understand how it works and what it needs to stay healthy. In this chapter, we will look at some basic aspects of human physiology and explain how they relate to self-healing.

The central nervous system, consisting of the brain and spinal cord, is responsible for controlling most bodily functions. It receives and interprets information from our environment and our inner self and sends commands to the rest of the body. The quality of this communication has a direct impact on our health and well-being.

Our cardiovascular system, the heart, blood vessels, and blood, is responsible for distributing oxygen and nutrients to our cells and eliminating waste products. A well-functioning cardiovascular system is essential for self-healing.

Our immune system protects us from diseases by recognizing and fighting foreign substances and microorganisms. It also plays a key role in the repair and regeneration of tissues.

Our digestive organs are responsible for breaking down food and absorbing the nutrients it contains. They also eliminate waste products. Healthy digestion is important to provide our body with the resources it needs to heal itself.

Our muscles and bones allow us to move and protect our internal organs. They also play an important role in maintaining our balance and stability.

In the following chapters, we will look at how we can support these systems through healthy eating, physical activity, adequate sleep, stress management, and other strategies. However, the first step in this journey is to develop an awareness of our body and its needs.

We hope this guide will help you discover and improve your ability to self-heal. Remember that you are the main player in your health journey and that you have the potential to change your life in a positive way.

Get ready for an exciting and enriching journey. It's time to take control of your health and discover the wonderful power of self-healing. Heal yourself!

Chapter 3: Healthy Eating: Food for Healing

Our diet is one of the most important factors in our health and well-being. The food we eat provides the raw materials our body needs to perform its multiple functions. It can either contribute to healing or promote disease.

In this chapter, we will look at the basics of a healthy diet and provide concrete tips and strategies for a nutrient-dense, balanced diet. In doing so, we will pay special attention to foods that support the body's self-healing processes.

Basically, a healthy diet consists of a variety of wholesome, unprocessed foods. Fruits and vegetables should make up the majority of our diet, as they are rich in vitamins, minerals, fiber, and antioxidants that help prevent and treat disease.

Whole grains, legumes, nuts and seeds provide complex carbohydrates, proteins, and healthy fats needed to provide energy and build and repair tissues. They also contain a lot of micronutrients and fiber, which contribute to overall health.

Fish and seafood are excellent sources of omega-3 fatty acids, which are important for brain function and have anti-inflammatory properties. They also contain many other nutrients such as iodine and
Vitamin D.

Meat and dairy products can be consumed in moderation, but they should not make up the main part of our diet. It is important to pay attention to the quality of these products and, if possible, give preference to organic and grass-fed products.

Sugar, refined carbohydrates and processed foods should be avoided as much as possible, as they are low in nutrients and can contribute to health problems such as obesity, type 2 diabetes and heart disease.

Water is another important aspect of our diet. It is involved in almost all bodily functions and is essential for self-healing. It is important to stay hydrated and limit alcoholic and sugary drinks.

It is also important to pay attention to your individual needs and preferences and choose a diet that you can maintain in the long term. It is better to make slow and sustained changes than to follow radical diets that are difficult to maintain.

In the next chapters, we will dive deeper into the different aspects of self-healing, from exercise and fitness to mental clarity and emotional balance to sleep and recovery. The path to health is a holistic process, and every decision you make will bring you one step closer to your goal. Heal yourself! Choosing the right diet is an art in itself. In our modern world, access to food from all over the world has never been easier. However, with this diversity comes a flood of information, opinions, and diet trends that can be confusing. Below, we'll explore some basic principles of a healthy diet to shed some light on this.

Nutritional basics: macronutrients and micronutrients

Food provides nutrients that our body needs to perform its functions. These nutrients can be broadly divided into two categories: macronutrients and micronutrients.

Macronutrients are nutrients that we need in large quantities and that provide energy. They include proteins, carbohydrates and fats.

1. **Proteins** are the building blocks of our body. They are necessary for the growth and repair of tissues, the production of hormones and enzymes, and many other functions. Good sources of protein include meat, fish, eggs, dairy products, legumes, nuts and seeds.

2. **Carbohydrates** are our main source of energy. They are converted into glucose, which is used as fuel by our cells. Carbohydrates are found in foods such as fruits, vegetables, whole grains, and legumes.

3. **Fats** are a concentrated source of energy and are necessary for the absorption of fat-soluble vitamins (A, D, E, K), the production of hormones and the health of skin and hair. Good sources of fat include avocados, nuts, seeds, olive oil, fish, and some meats.

Micronutrients are nutrients that we need in smaller amounts, but they are just as important for our health. They include vitamins and minerals that are involved in almost all bodily functions.

The plate of health

A helpful tool for designing healthy meals is the "Plate of Health". Imagine that your plate is divided into four parts. Fill half of the plate with vegetables, a quarter with proteins, and a quarter with whole grains or starchy vegetables. Add a serving of healthy fats and drink plenty of water. Fruits can be enjoyed as a dessert or snack between meals.

Intuitive nutrition

Another important aspect of a healthy diet is intuitive nutrition. This approach emphasizes listening to the internal hunger signals and awareness of the emotional and physical impact of our food choices. Intuitive nutrition teaches us to respect our bodies and see food as a source of nutrients and enjoyment, rather than as an enemy in a constant battle to control weight.

In summary, a healthy diet should be diverse, nutritious and enjoyable. It should provide us with the necessary nutrients, make us feel full and satisfied, and allow us to live our lives to the fullest.

In the next chapters, we will look at other aspects of self-healing, such as exercise, stress management, sleep, and social relationships. We will also look at the role of mental and emotional health in healing and health. The path to health is a journey, and this guide is your compass. Get ready for a full and healthy life. Heal yourself!

Chapter 4: Exercise as Medicine: The Role of Physical Activity in Self-Healing

Exercise is another pillar of self-healing and health. Not only does it help with weight control, but it also has numerous health benefits that go beyond physical fitness.

Why is exercise important?

Regular physical activity can reduce the risk of many chronic diseases such as heart disease, diabetes, some cancers, arthritis and osteoporosis. It also contributes to mental health by reducing the risk of depression and anxiety and improving overall well-being.

Exercise increases blood flow, which improves the transport of nutrients and oxygen to our cells and promotes the elimination of waste products. It also stimulates the immune system, improves digestion and sleep, and increases energy.

How much and what kind of exercise?

The World Health Organization recommends at least 150 minutes of moderate exercise or 75 minutes of vigorous exercise per week, or a combination of both. In addition, muscle-strengthening activities should be carried out twice a week.

However, it is important to emphasize that every movement counts and is useful. If you're just starting out, or if you're unable to meet these recommendations for health reasons, it's okay. Start where you are and gradually increase your activity.

There are many different types of exercises, and the best ones are the ones you can enjoy and do regularly. It can be helpful to combine a variety of activities to address different aspects of fitness:

1. **Aerobic exercise** improves cardiovascular health and endurance. Examples include fast walking, running, cycling, swimming, dancing, and many team sports.

2. **Strength training** improves muscle strength and mass, metabolism and bone health. It can be done with weights, resistance bands, or your own body weight (as in yoga or pilates).

3. **Flexibility and balance exercises** help prevent injuries and improve mobility and overall quality of life. They are an important part of disciplines such as yoga and tai chi, but can also be performed as practices in their own right.

Overcoming barriers

It's common to run into obstacles when you're trying to incorporate more exercise into your life. Here are some tips on how to overcome them:

1. **Lack of time**: Plan your workouts in advance and treat them like any other important appointment. Short workouts during the day can be just as effective as longer sessions. Take advantage of breaks and waiting times for short activities such as walks or stretching exercises.

2. **Lack of motivation**: Set realistic goals and track your progress. Find activities you enjoy and vary your workout to avoid boredom. Work with a friend or group, or consider a personal trainer or coach.

3. **Physical discomfort or health problems**: Talk to your doctor before starting any new exercise program, especially if you have chronic illnesses or have been inactive for a long time. Choose activities that fit your skills and needs. A physical therapist or a qualified fitness trainer can help you create a safe and effective program.

In conclusion, exercise plays a vital role in promoting self-healing and maintaining health. It is a simple and effective medicine that is accessible to everyone. Take the first step and discover the joy and benefits of physical activity. Heal yourself!

The Role of Exercise in Mental Health

It is equally important to highlight the role of exercise in promoting mental health. Physical activity has been shown to improve mood, reduce stress, anxiety, and depression, improve sleep quality, and even boost memory and cognitive function. Exercise is thought to achieve these effects in part by releasing endorphins (the so-called "happiness hormones") and promoting neurogenesis (the formation of new nerve cells) in the brain.

Also, movement can be a form of meditation in motion, especially when combined with mindfulness. Mindful movement, such as yoga or tai chi, can help draw attention to the present moment, calm the mind, and promote a sense of inner peace and balance.

Movement and connection

Exercise can also be a way to connect with other people and encourage social support and belonging. This can be done by participating in team sports, fitness classes, or simply by walking or cycling with friends or family members. In addition, contact with nature through outdoor activities, such as hiking or gardening, can promote a sense of connection and appreciation for the natural world, which also contributes to mental health and well-being.

Building an exercise routine

It can be helpful to create a regular exercise plan to facilitate compliance. Try to make exercise an integral part of your daily routine, just as you eat and sleep. It can be helpful to try exercise at different times of the day to see what works best for you: Some people find that they have more energy to exercise in the morning, while others prefer to exercise in the evening to relieve the stress of the day.

Do not forget that it is important to listen to your body and give yourself time to rest and regenerate. Overtraining can lead to injury and exhaustion and is ultimately counterproductive. Just as important as the movement itself is the time you give yourself to recover from it.

Result

Exercise is a powerful tool for self-healing and health promotion. It is a gift we can give to ourselves and others, an investment in our health and quality of life that pays off over time. Take the first step today and discover the joys and benefits of physical activity. Heal yourself!

Chapter 5: Stress Management: The Art of Finding Calm in the Midst of the Storm

Stress is an inescapable part of modern life. Although some degree of stress can be healthy and even beneficial, spurring us on and helping us face challenges, chronic or excessive stress can cause serious health problems and affect our overall well-being. That's why it's important to develop effective stress management strategies.

What is stress?

Stress is our body's way of responding to any kind of requirement or threat. When we feel threatened, our nervous system sets in motion a series of chemical reactions known as the "fight-or-flight" response. This response prepares our bodies to either fight or flee by increasing heart rate, blood pressure, and blood sugar levels, as well as sharpening our senses.

This response was useful in early human history, when the threats were mainly physical (such as the attack of a predator). However, in today's world, the threats are mostly psychological (such as deadline pressures or financial worries), and the "fight-or-flight" response can do more harm than good.

The effects of chronic stress

Chronic stress can lead to a variety of health problems, including heart disease, diabetes, sleep disorders, digestive problems, skin conditions, mental health problems (such as depression and anxiety), and a weakened immune system. It can also lead to unhealthy behaviors such as overeating, smoking, alcohol and drug use, and social isolation.

Stress management strategies

There are many effective strategies for managing stress, and what works for one person may not work for another. Here are some general strategies:

1. **Mindfulness practice**: Mindfulness means focusing attention on the present moment and accepting the experiences of the moment without judgment. Mindfulness meditation, yoga, and tai chi are examples of practices that promote mindfulness.

2. **Deep Breathing and Relaxation Techniques**: Deep breathing, progressive muscle relaxation, biofeedback, and guided imagery are techniques that can help calm the "fight-or-flight" state and promote a more relaxed state.

3. **Exercise**: As mentioned earlier, exercise is an effective way to manage stress. It can help reduce stress hormones, improve mood, and promote an overall sense of well-being.

4. **Healthy eating**: A healthy diet can help strengthen the body and mind and improve resistance to stress.

5. **Social support**: Social support can cushion stress and promote a sense of belonging and shared understanding. This can be achieved through friendships, family, support groups, or therapeutic support.

6. **Get enough sleep**: Sleep is an important time for the body and mind to recover and regenerate. A lack of sleep can increase the body's stress response and impair the ability to cope with stress.

It's important that you take a holistic approach to stress management that is tailored to your specific needs and circumstances. Remember that it's okay to ask for help and seek support if you need it.

Create a customized stress management plan

One of the most effective ways to manage stress is to create an individualized stress management plan. This plan should be specific, measurable, achievable, relevant, and time-bound – what is commonly known as SMART goals. Here are some steps that might help you create your personal stress management plan:

1. **Identify your stress triggers**: The first step to managing stress is to recognize what triggers your stress. These can be external factors such as workload, relationship problems or financial worries, but also internal factors such as perfectionism, negative thinking or high self-demands.

2. **Choose your stress management strategies**: Decide which strategies you want to use to manage your stress. You may need to try and adjust different strategies until you figure out what works best for you.

3. **Create an action plan**: Set specific goals and write an action plan that indicates when and how you will implement your stress management strategies. Try to make your goals as specific and realistic as possible.

4. **Evaluate and adjust your plan**: Regularly review your progress and adjust your plan if necessary. Be lenient with yourself if you don't reach your goal, and see every setback as an opportunity to learn and grow.

Healing effects of leisure and hobbies

Another effective stress management strategy is to set aside time for leisure activities and hobbies on a regular basis. Hobbies can provide a welcome distraction from stressful situations and help relax the mind and recharge your batteries. They can also provide a sense of accomplishment and satisfaction and help boost self-esteem and self-efficacy.

Hobbies can be as diverse as the people who practice them. It can be creative activities such as painting, making music or writing, physical activities such as dancing, hiking or gardening, or mental activities such as reading, playing chess or solving puzzles. It is important that you choose activities that you enjoy and that you find enriching and fulfilling.

Result

Stress management is a vital skill in our hectic and often overwhelming world. By learning and practicing effective stress management strategies, we can strengthen our resilience, improve our quality of life, and promote well-being. Take the first step and start implementing your personal stress management plan today. Heal yourself!

Chapter 5: The Power of Positive Relationships

One of the most basic human needs is the need for connection and belonging. Positive relationships with other people are a crucial factor in our well-being and quality of life. They provide support and encouragement, enrich our lives with joy and satisfaction, help us manage stress and boost our self-esteem.

Social support and health

There are numerous studies that prove the link between social support and health. People who have strong social networks and supportive relationships tend to have better mental and physical health and live longer. They have a lower risk of a variety of diseases, including heart disease, depression, and anxiety, and they recover faster from illness and injury.

Social support can come in many forms: it can be emotional (such as affection, affection, or encouragement), informational (such as advice or information), material (such as financial help or practical support), or socially-inclusive (such as a sense of belonging to a community or group).

Building and maintaining positive relationships

Building and maintaining positive relationships takes time, energy, and dedication. Here are some tips that might help you with this:

1. **Be attentive and present**: When spending time with other people, be fully present and pay attention to their words, feelings, and needs. Try to listen without judgment and show genuine interest and compassion.

2. **Communicate openly and honestly**: Share your thoughts, feelings, and needs openly and honestly with others, and encourage them to do the same. Constructive communication can clear up misunderstandings, resolve conflicts, and strengthen the connection.

3. **Show appreciation**: Show your appreciation for the people in your life through words and deeds. A simple thank you, a loving gesture, or a compliment can make a big difference.

4. **Set healthy boundaries**: Respect your own needs and boundaries and those of others. It's okay to say no, take time for yourself, and ask for support when you need it.

The importance of self-love

Ultimately, the strongest and healthiest relationships are those based on love and respect for oneself. When we love and accept ourselves as we are, we are better able to love and accept others as they are. Self-love also promotes our emotional health and resilience and allows us to better cope with stress and difficulties.

Remember: healing starts from within. Take time to take care of yourself, be patient with yourself, and celebrate your progress and successes. They are worth it!

Chapter 7: Nature's Healing Power

Nature has an amazing ability to soothe, refresh and inspire us. Whether we're taking a walk in the woods, watching a sunset, or just breathing in the fresh air, nature can help us ground ourselves and regain our balance. In this chapter, we will explore the healing effects of nature and some ways you can use them in your own life.

The benefits of nature for body and mind

Science has shown that contact with nature has a variety of health benefits. For example:

- **Improve mental health**: Experiencing nature can help reduce anxiety and depression, improve well-being, and increase life satisfaction. They can also promote creativity and focus and help reduce stress.

- **Physical Health Promotion**: Nature encourages physical activity and exercise, which can lead to improved overall health, reduced risk of chronic disease, and improved quality of life. It can also strengthen the immune system and improve sleep quality.

- **Improving social connections**: Shared nature experiences can help strengthen relationships, foster a sense of community, and improve social skills.

Experience nature in your everyday life

There are many different ways to integrate nature into your everyday life. Here are some suggestions:

1. **Make time for an outdoor walk**: A daily outdoor walk, whether in the park, in the woods, or just in your neighborhood, can help you relax, refresh yourself, and clear your mind.

2. **Cultivate plants in your home or garden**: Caring for plants can be a satisfying and calming activity that helps you connect with nature even when you're not outdoors.

3. **Engage in outdoor activities**: Hiking, biking, swimming, gardening, or just having an outdoor picnic can help you reap the benefits of nature while staying physically active.

4. **Take time to admire nature**: watch birds, admire flowers, look up at the sky and let your senses be fascinated by the beauty and diversity of nature.

Remember that it is important to treat nature with respect and gratitude. Nature is a precious resource that has a lot to offer us, and it is our responsibility to protect and preserve it for future generations.

Chapter 8: The Mental Healing Power: Healing by the Spirit

Our mind and psyche play a crucial role in our well-being and our ability to heal ourselves. In this chapter we will look at how mental and emotional aspects affect our health and how we can use them to promote self-healing.

1. The power of thoughts: Our thoughts have a direct impact on our emotions, our behavior, and ultimately our physical state. Negative thoughts and emotional distress can affect our body and increase the risk of disease. By consciously acquiring positive thoughts and an optimistic point of view, we can strengthen our psyche and activate our self-healing powers.

2. Stress management: Stress is a natural part of life, but chronic stress can lead to a variety of health problems. The ability to manage and manage stress is therefore crucial for our self-healing. In this chapter we will learn about different techniques and strategies for coping with stress, such as relaxation exercises, breathing techniques, meditation and mindfulness.

3. Emotional balance: Emotional imbalances can affect our body and affect our health. By dealing with our own emotions, accepting them and dealing with them appropriately, we can restore our emotional balance and promote our self-healing. In this chapter we will learn methods for regulating emotions and promoting positive emotions.

4. The importance of social support: Relationships and social connections play an important role in our well-being and health. A strong social network and supportive relationships can strengthen our resilience and help us cope with difficult times. In this chapter, we will explore the importance of social support and the healing power of community.

5. The role of spirituality: Spirituality can take different forms and be different for each person. Regardless of religious beliefs, spirituality can be a source of inspiration, hope, and empowerment. We will explore the importance of mindfulness, meditation, prayer or other spiritual practices for furthering our self-healing powers.

6. Psychotherapy and counseling: Sometimes it is helpful to seek professional support to heal our psyche and promote our self-healing. In this chapter we will learn about different psychotherapeutic approaches and counseling methods that can help us cope with emotional challenges and promote our mental health.

By healing our psyche and strengthening our mental health, we can activate our self-healing powers and promote our health on a holistic level. The mind and body are closely linked, and a holistic approach to self-healing takes into account both physical and psychological aspects.

Embark on a journey to explore your psyche and activate your self-healing powers. Learn to pay attention to your thoughts and emotions and make positive changes that will help you improve your health and well-being. The power of the psyche is in your hands, use it to heal yourself and live a full life of health and well-being.

Please note that this guide is not intended as a substitute for professional medical advice or treatment. If you have any health problems, please consult a qualified doctor or therapist.

Chapter 9: Nutrition and physical health

It is well known that a healthy diet and regular physical activity are essential components of a healthy life. But how exactly do these aspects affect our health and how can we heal ourselves by paying attention to them? In this chapter, we will dive deeper into these topics.

The Role of Nutrition in Healing

Our diet plays an essential role in the functioning of our body and directly affects our health. A balanced diet provides the body with the necessary nutrients it needs for energy production, growth, repair and maintenance of all bodily functions.

Vitamins and minerals that we get from a varied and balanced diet are crucial for strengthening our immune system and for preventing and fighting diseases. In addition, the type of food we eat has a direct impact on our mood and overall well-being.

Physical activity as a healing factor

Regular physical activity has a variety of health benefits. It improves cardiovascular health, strengthens muscles, promotes bone health, and supports weight control. In addition, exercise helps to improve our mood and reduce anxiety and stress.

Equally important, regular physical activity can reduce the risk of a number of diseases, including heart disease, stroke, type 2 diabetes, certain cancers, and osteoporosis.

Steps to a healthy diet and physical activity

A healthy diet and physical activity are achievable goals. Here are some steps that might inspire you to do so:

1. **Choose a variety of foods**: Try to eat a variety of foods from all food groups to ensure you're getting a wide range of nutrients.

2. **Eat plenty of fruits and vegetables**: Fruits and vegetables are rich in vitamins, minerals, and fiber and should be a big part of your diet.

3. **Stay hydrated**: Drink enough water throughout the day to keep your body hydrated and support all of its functions.

4. **Incorporate exercise into your daily routine**: Find activities that you enjoy and try to incorporate them into your daily routine on a regular basis. It could be as simple as taking a daily walk, dancing to your favorite music, or taking a weekly yoga class.

Do not forget that changes in lifestyle habits take time. Be patient with yourself and celebrate every little progress on your path to health and healing.

Chapter 10: The Power of Positive Thoughts

Our thoughts have a remarkable effect on our well-being and our ability to heal ourselves. Negative thoughts and beliefs can burden us, increase stress and anxiety and block our self-healing powers. On the other hand, positive thoughts and an optimistic mindset can improve our mood, reduce stress, and strengthen our ability to recover and heal ourselves.

The effects of negative thoughts

Negative thoughts and beliefs can lead to a vicious cycle that affects our health and well-being. When we focus on negative thoughts, we increase our fears, doubts, and worries. This can lead to stress, which in turn affects our physical and mental health.

Negative thoughts can also affect our perception and interpretation of events. We tend to focus on the negative and overlook positive aspects. This can affect our mood and overall well-being and hinder our ability to self-heal.

Interestingly, studies have shown that negative thoughts and pessimism can weaken the immune system. Chronic stress caused by negative thoughts leads to an increase in stress hormones such as cortisol, which can suppress the immune system. As a result, we are more susceptible to illness and may have a longer recovery time.

Negative thoughts can also lead to a lack of motivation and agency. When we convince ourselves that we are not able to heal ourselves, we put less effort into it and do not use the full potential of our self-healing powers.

The Power of Positive Thoughts

Positive thoughts and an optimistic mindset, on the other hand, can strengthen our self-healing powers. By focusing on the positive and believing in our ability to recover, we can increase our motivation and determination. Positive thoughts can reduce stress, improve our mood, and promote our physical and mental health.

Studies have shown that a positive mindset is associated with improved immune function, faster recovery from disease, and a better quality of life. People with an optimistic attitude often have higher levels of self-confidence and are better able to cope with stress.

Interestingly, positive thoughts can also affect brain activity. Researchers have found that practicing positive thoughts and affirmations increases activity in the areas of the brain associated with reward, motivation, and positive emotions. By fostering this positive brain activity, we can change our thought patterns and arrive at a more optimistic mindset.

Positive thoughts can also lead to better management of stress. By focusing on the positive and staying optimistic, we can better manage stressful situations and reduce negative effects on our health. A positive mindset helps us find solutions and tackle challenges with confidence.

Practices for positive thoughts

There are several practices that can help you cultivate positive thoughts and promote an optimistic mindset:

1. **Mindfulness**: Mindfulness means perceiving the present moment consciously and without judgment. By being mindful, you can identify and let go of negative thoughts and instead focus on the positive and the present. You can practice mindfulness meditation or breathing exercises to sharpen your attention and calm your thoughts.

2. **Positive Affirmations**: Use positive statements and affirmations to overcome negative self-talk and encourage yourself. Repeat positive statements such as "I am strong and capable" or "I have the ability to heal myself" on a daily basis. Write down these affirmations and read them regularly to positively influence your subconscious mind.

3. **Gratitude**: Take time each day to be grateful. Write down three things you're grateful for or share with someone. The practice of gratitude can help shift the focus to the positive and encourage a positive mindset. You can keep a gratitude journal or just consciously think about what you are grateful for every day.

4. **Visualization**: Imagine in your mind how you feel healthy and healed. Visualize your body and mind in a state of well-being. Vividly imagine how you will achieve your goals and restore your health. This technique can help amplify positive thoughts and emotions and activate your self-healing powers.

5. **Dealing with negative thoughts**: Learn to recognize and question negative thoughts. Ask yourself if these thoughts are really true and helpful. Often, negative thoughts are distorted and not objective. Make an effort to replace these negative thoughts with positive and realistic thoughts.

6. **Environment and Relationships**: Surround yourself with positive people and a supportive environment. Exchanging positive thoughts and interacting with optimistic people can be contagious and affect your own way of thinking. Avoid negative influences, whether in the form of people or media, and consciously look for inspiring and positive sources.

By incorporating these practices into your daily routine and focusing on positive thoughts and an optimistic mindset, you can support your ability to self-heal and increase your well-being.

Interestingly, studies have shown that people with a positive mindset have a longer life expectancy and are less likely to suffer from chronic diseases. Positive thoughts can help reduce stress, boost the immune system, and improve overall quality of life.

It's important to note that positive thoughts alone can't do miracles, but they can have a significant impact on our attitudes, behaviors, and health. By consciously choosing positive thoughts and cultivating your mindset, you can support yourself on the path to self-healing.

Remember that it is normal to have occasional negative thoughts. The key is to recognize these thoughts and actively work to replace them with positive and constructive thoughts. Over time and with continuous practice, you can change your thought patterns and develop a positive and optimistic mindset that supports your health and self-healing powers.

Chapter 11: Naturopathy: Traditional Healing Methods

Naturopathy is a branch of medicine based on the earth's natural resources and has been used for thousands of years. Many cultures around the world have developed their own traditional healing methods based on plants, herbs, minerals and other natural substances. In this chapter, we will look at some of the most well-known traditional healing methods in naturopathy and explore their application to self-healing.

Healing herbs and plants

Herbs and plants have long been known for their healing properties. In naturopathy, they are used to treat various ailments and promote health. Each plant has its own specific active ingredients and applications. Here are some well-known medicinal plants and their uses:

- Chamomile: Chamomile has anti-inflammatory and soothing properties. It is often used to relieve gastrointestinal discomfort, sleep disorders and skin problems.

- St. John's wort: St. John's wort is used to treat mild to moderate depression. It has mood-enhancing properties and can also be helpful for nervousness and sleep disorders.

- Ginger: Ginger has anti-inflammatory and digestive properties. It is often used for indigestion, nausea and inflammation.

- Echinacea: Echinacea is used to support the immune system and can increase resistance to infections. It is often used for colds, flu and other infectious diseases.

- Lavender: Lavender has calming and relaxing properties. It is often used to relieve stress, anxiety and insomnia.

These are just a few examples of medicinal plants used in naturopathy. It is important to find out about the correct use and dosage, and to consult a professional if necessary.

Acupuncture

Acupuncture is a traditional Chinese healing method in which fine needles are inserted at specific points on the body. It is believed that these points are connected to energy pathways in the body and that stimulation of these points can balance and promote the flow of energy in the body. Acupuncture is used to treat various conditions, including pain, stress, sleep disorders, and digestive problems. It is important to consult a qualified acupuncturist who has in-depth knowledge and experience.

Ayurveda

Ayurveda is a traditional Indian healing system based on a holistic view of the body and the

Health based. It is based on the balance of body, mind and soul. Various methods are used in Ayurvedic medicine, including herbal medicine, nutrition, massage, yoga, and meditation. The aim is to restore the balance of individual constitutional types (doshas) and to support the body's self-healing powers.

Homeopathy

Homeopathy is an alternative healing method based on the principle of "like is cured with like". Homeopathic remedies are made from natural substances and are used in high dilution. It is believed that these remedies stimulate the body's self-healing powers and restore energetic balance. A homeopathic doctor can take into account the individual symptoms and personal constitution in order to select the appropriate homeopathic remedy.

These traditional healing methods of naturopathy are often complementary to conventional medicine and can be a valuable addition. It is important to find out about the application and possible interactions, as well as to consult a qualified professional. Naturopathy offers a wide range of approaches to support self-healing and promote health naturally.

The world of naturopathy is rich and there are many more traditional healing methods and approaches. Every person is unique, and what works for one may not work for another. Experiment, educate yourself, and find the approaches that suit you best. By incorporating these traditional healing methods, you can further strengthen your ability to self-heal and promote your well-being in a natural way.

In naturopathy, nutrition also plays a central role. A healthy and balanced diet is crucial for self-healing and general well-being. By eating natural, unprocessed foods, we provide our body with important nutrients it needs to heal itself.

It is advisable to include a variety of fresh fruits and vegetables in the diet. These are rich in vitamins, minerals, and antioxidants that can protect the body from free radical damage. Preferably, choose organically grown foods to minimize the use of pesticides and other chemicals.

Whole grains such as oatmeal, whole grain bread, and brown rice should be given preference over refined grain products. They contain fiber, which can aid digestion and stabilize blood sugar levels.

Proteins are important for building and repairing tissue. Choose lean meats, fish, eggs, legumes, and plant-based protein sources such as tofu or quinoa. Fish is particularly rich in omega-3 fatty acids, which may have anti-inflammatory properties.

Healthy fats such as olive oil, nuts and avocado should also be incorporated into the diet. They provide important essential fatty acids that are important for skin, brain and heart health.

The consumption of sugary drinks and processed foods should be minimized. These often contain high amounts of added sugars, preservatives, and artificial ingredients that can put a strain on the body. Instead, you should prefer fresh, home-cooked food.

Naturopathy also includes the use of various healing methods such as massages, aromatherapy, hydrotherapy and medicinal plants. These methods can help restore balance in the body, reduce stress, and support self-healing powers.

Regular physical activity is also an important part of naturopathy. Exercise promotes blood circulation, strengthens the immune system and improves mood. Choose an activity that you enjoy, whether it's yoga, jogging, swimming, or dancing, and incorporate it into your daily routine on a regular basis.

Naturopathy offers a holistic view of health and promotes self-healing in a natural way. By providing our body with the right nutrients, moving it around, and using various healing methods, we can support our health and well-being.

It is important to note that naturopathy is not used as a substitute for school medicine.

medical care should be considered. In the event of serious health problems, it is advisable to consult a qualified professional and follow a holistic treatment that takes into account both conventional and naturopathic approaches.

In the following chapters, we will look at other aspects of self-healing, including the importance of mindfulness and spirituality, relationships and social life, stress management and prevention. By taking a holistic approach to our health and integrating different approaches, we can strengthen our ability to self-heal and live a healthy and fulfilling life.

Chapter 12: Mindfulness and Spirituality: The Importance of Faith and Spirit

In our hectic and stressful world, it is important to find moments of silence and inner peace. Mindfulness and spirituality offer opportunities to connect with a deeper level of our being and strengthen the self-healing powers. In this chapter, we will explore the importance of mindfulness and spirituality for our health and well-being.

Mindfulness: Living consciously in the here and now

Mindfulness means living consciously in the present moment and accepting the experiences without judgment. It's about calming the mind and focusing on the here and now. Through mindfulness practices such as meditation, breathing exercises, and conscious eating, we can detach ourselves from stressful thoughts and external distractions.

Studies have shown that mindfulness has numerous positive effects on our health. It can reduce stress, improve sleep quality, promote emotional balance and strengthen the immune system. By consciously focusing on the present moment, we can activate our self-healing powers and support our health.

Spirituality: The connection to the higher

Spirituality refers to the belief in a higher power or consciousness that transcends us. It can take different forms, depending on individual beliefs and traditions. Spirituality offers a way to find meaning and purpose in our lives and connect with something bigger.

Believing in something higher can bring a deep inner peace and serenity. It can help us deal with challenges, find hope, and clarify our own values and priorities. Through spiritual practices such as prayer, meditation, closeness to nature and rituals, we can connect with our inner spiritual nature.

Studies have shown that spiritual people often have better mental health and are better able to cope with stress. Believing in something higher can be a source of comfort, support, and trust, especially in difficult times.

The connection between mindfulness and spirituality

Mindfulness and spirituality can be closely related. By living mindfully, we can connect more consciously with our spiritual nature and perceive the experiences of the present moment more intensely. Through mindfulness practices, we can calm our minds and deepen our spiritual connection.

Mindfulness can also help clarify our spiritual beliefs and recognize our values. By focusing on our inner voice and intuition, we can better align ourselves with our faith and spirituality.

The Importance of Faith and Spirit for Self-Healing

Faith and the Spirit play an important role in self-healing. When we firmly believe that we have the ability to heal ourselves, we strengthen our inner conviction and optimism. The mind can mobilize an amazing power of healing and support the body in its self-healing process.

Stress and negative thoughts can put a strain on the body and impair its self-healing powers. By focusing on positive thoughts, affirmations, and visualizations, we can foster a positive mental attitude and support the healing process.

The combination of mindfulness, spirituality and faith can help us strengthen our health and well-being on all levels. By consciously connecting with our inner self and a higher power, we can activate the self-healing powers and live a full and healthy life.

Awareness of mindfulness and spirituality can be developed in different ways. Here are some practices and approaches that can help you strengthen your mindfulness and deepen your spiritual connection:

1. Meditation: The practice of meditation can help you calm your mind and immerse yourself in the present moment. Sit in a quiet place, close your eyes, and focus on your breath or a specific focus, such as a mantra or image. Let your thoughts pass by without holding on to them and return to your focus again and again.

2. Closeness to nature: Spend time in nature and be inspired by its beauty and tranquility. Go for a walk, go hiking or just sit in a park and consciously perceive your surroundings. Pay attention to the sounds, smells and textures around you and feel the connection to nature.

3. Prayer: If you are religious, prayers can be an important part of your spiritual practice. Take time to pray and express your gratitude, wishes, and concerns. Prayer can help you strengthen your connection to a higher power and let go of your inner worries and fears.

4. Write a journal: Keep a journal to record your thoughts, feelings, and insights. Write about your spiritual experiences, your desires and goals, or reflect on events in your life. Journaling can help you organize your thoughts, hear your inner voice, and track your spiritual development.

5. Community: Look for communities or groups that deal with mindfulness and spirituality. Sharing with like-minded people can help you gain new perspectives, inspire each other, and deepen your practice. Take part in meditation groups, spiritual retreats or workshops to gain new experiences and expand your knowledge.

6. Self-reflection: Take regular time for self-reflection and introspection. Sit in a quiet room and consciously take time to reflect on your thoughts, feelings, and life experiences. Ask yourself questions like: What is really important to me in life? What brings me joy and fulfillment? How can I further deepen my spiritual practice?

By incorporating these practices into your everyday life and consciously living mindfully and spiritually, you can strengthen your ability to self-heal. Be patient and give yourself the time to evolve and explore your spiritual journey.

Chapter 13: Preventive measures: prevention is better than cure.

In this chapter, we will take an in-depth look at the topic of preventive measures and explain how prevention can make a significant contribution to self-healing. Prevention aims to prevent diseases before they arise and to identify risk factors in order to be able to intervene in time. Prevention is a central part of a healthy and balanced lifestyle.

1. Regular health check-ups: Regular visits to the doctor and comprehensive health check-ups are of great importance to detect potential health problems at an early stage. These examinations include blood tests, cholesterol measurements, blood pressure checks, and targeted examinations for the early detection of diseases such as cancer. Regular examinations can reduce the risk of serious illness and ensure timely treatment.

2. Healthy diet: A balanced and nutritious diet is of great importance to prevent diseases. A healthy diet rich in fruits, vegetables, whole grains, lean protein and healthy fats provides the body with the necessary nutrients, strengthens the immune system and protects against various diseases such as heart disease, diabetes and obesity. Make sure you have a varied and balanced diet that meets your individual needs and preferences.

3. Physical activity: Regular physical activity is an important part of disease prevention. By exercising regularly, you will not only strengthen your cardiovascular system, but also improve your physical fitness, increase your energy and reduce the risk of chronic diseases such as diabetes, heart disease and certain types of cancer. Find activities that you enjoy and can be integrated into your daily routine, whether it's walking, jogging, swimming or cycling.

4. Stress management: Chronic stress can have a negative impact on health and increase the risk of heart disease, depression and other diseases. Therefore, it is important to learn effective stress management techniques and integrate them into everyday life. These include relaxation exercises such as meditation, yoga, breathing techniques, regular breaks, and promoting a balanced lifestyle.

5. Not smoking: Smoking is one of the leading causes of serious diseases such as lung cancer, heart disease, and respiratory diseases. To reduce your risk of these diseases, it is advisable to quit smoking or not to start. If necessary, seek support to successfully implement smoking cessation.

6. Alcohol consumption: Excessive alcohol consumption can cause serious health problems, including liver disease, cancer, cardiovascular disease, and mental disorders. Follow the recommended guidelines for moderate alcohol consumption and be aware of the effects of alcohol on your body and health.

7. Sleep hygiene: Adequate and quality sleep is essential for the regeneration and self-healing of the body. Maintain good sleep hygiene by maintaining a regular bedtime, creating a quiet and dark place to sleep, and practicing relaxation techniques before bed.

8. Healthy environment: Surround yourself with a healthy environment that is free of pollutants, pollutants and allergens. Pay attention to good air quality, avoid excessive pollution pollution and pay attention to a safe and clean living and working environment.

By taking preventive measures, you can reduce the risk of disease and promote your health and well-being in the long term. Remember that prevention is a continuous process and is made up of various lifestyle factors. Be proactive and invest in your health by taking the necessary steps to prevent disease.

Chapter 14: The Power of **Self-Reflection: The Healing Power of Inner Dialogue**

Our inner dialogue, the way we talk to ourselves and perceive our thoughts, plays a crucial role in our well-being and our ability to self-heal. In this chapter we will look at how we can consciously use inner dialogue to promote our mental health and activate our self-healing powers.

1. Self-confidence and self-acceptance: A positive and healthy relationship with oneself is an important part of self-healing. By getting to know ourselves better and accepting ourselves, we can create a deeper connection to our inner being and develop a loving attitude towards ourselves.

2. The power of affirmations: Affirmations are positive statements that we consciously repeat to strengthen our thoughts and beliefs. By using positive affirmations, we can program our subconscious mind in a healthy and healing way. We will learn how to formulate effective affirmations and integrate them into everyday life.

3. Transform the inner critic: Often we have an inner critic who constantly evaluates us negatively and pulls us down. In this chapter we will learn how to identify and transform our inner critic. We will learn techniques for realigning negative thought patterns and learn to treat ourselves more compassionately and lovingly.

4. The art of self-reflection: Self-reflection allows us to consciously engage with our thoughts, feelings, and actions. By taking time for self-reflection on a regular basis, we can understand ourselves better, identify our needs, and be more conscious of our actions. We will learn about different methods of self-reflection, such as keeping a diary, meditation or talking to a trusted person.

5. The power of visualization: Visualization is a powerful technique in which we consciously imagine positive images and scenarios in our minds. By practicing visualization regularly, we can align our subconscious mind with positive experiences and healing. We will learn how to effectively use visualization techniques to support self-healing.

6. The importance of self-care: Self-care is a central part of self-healing. In this chapter, we will learn how to lovingly care for ourselves by setting healthy boundaries, taking regular breaks, pampering ourselves with positive activities, and taking care of our physical, emotional, and mental well-being.

By consciously engaging with our inner dialogue and shaping it in a positive way, we can

we strengthen our mental health and activate our self-healing powers. The power of self-reflection allows us to use our inner voice as allies on our path to health and well-being.

Chapter 15: The Power of Self-Love: A Key to Wholeness and Healing

Self-love is an essential aspect of self-healing and well-being. In this chapter, we will explore the importance of self-love and explore ways to cultivate it in our lives. Self-love is not a selfish or narcissistic attitude, but a profound and unconditional acceptance and appreciation of our own being.

1. The importance of self-acceptance: Self-love begins with the complete acceptance of ourselves, including our strengths, weaknesses, and imperfections. We will explore how to free ourselves from self-criticism and self-judgments in order to treat ourselves with compassion and understanding.

2. Self-care as an expression of love: Self-love is also evident in our ability to take good care of ourselves and take care of our well-being. We will explore various aspects of self-care, such as physical health, emotional well-being, mental relaxation, and spiritual nourishment. It's about empowering ourselves and lovingly caring for ourselves.

3. Set boundaries and strengthen self-esteem: An important component of self-love is the ability to set healthy boundaries and strengthen our self-esteem. We will learn how to protect ourselves from being overwhelmed and exploited and how to value ourselves. By taking our own needs seriously and standing up for ourselves, we strengthen our self-esteem and self-love.

4. Forgiveness and letting go: Self-love also includes the willingness to forgive ourselves and let go of the past. We will realize that we all make mistakes and that this is a natural part of our growth. By forgiving ourselves and freeing ourselves from past burdens, we create space for healing and a loving relationship with ourselves.

5. The potential for self-transformation: Self-love is a process of personal transformation. We will explore the possibility of overcoming old beliefs, negative thought patterns and self-limiting beliefs and unleashing our full potential. Self-love encourages us to renew ourselves and consciously open ourselves to positive change.

6. Connecting with others: Self-love does not mean isolating oneself from others, but developing a healthy relationship with oneself and others. We will learn how to build loving and supportive relationships while maintaining our individual integrity. Finding a balance between self-love and connection enriches our lives and supports our healing journey.

By connecting with the power of self-love, we open ourselves to inner healing and wholeness. Self-love is the key to unleashing our self-healing potentials and living a fulfilled and authentic life. With every step we take on the path to self-love, we open up new opportunities for healing and personal growth.

Explore the power of self-love and let it blossom in your life. Give yourself the love, appreciation, and acceptance you deserve. You are valuable and lovable, just the way you are. In self-love you will find the source of wholeness and healing.

By embedding the power of self-love in our lives, we can experience a profound transformation. Here are other aspects of self-love that help us achieve wholeness and healing:

7. Self-awareness and self-expression: Self-love allows us to express ourselves confidently and clearly communicate our needs, desires, and limitations. We recognize our own values and stand by them. By finding our voice and being authentic, we strengthen our self-love and improve our relationships.

8. Gratitude and self-esteem: Self-love also involves the ability to develop gratitude for who we are and have. We learn to value ourselves for our strengths, talents and successes. By looking at ourselves with a loving gaze and acknowledging ourselves, we increase our self-esteem and self-love.

9. Self-reflection and personal growth: Self-love encourages us to reflect on ourselves and work on our personal growth. We take the time to get to know ourselves, understand our behavioral patterns, and question our ways of thinking. Through this self-reflection, we can heal old wounds and evolve.

10. Self-forgiveness and compassion: Self-love also involves the ability to forgive ourselves and be compassionate with ourselves. We recognize that we all make mistakes and that we can learn from them. By treating ourselves compassionately and forgiving ourselves, we break the cycle of self-criticism and allow ourselves inner peace.

11. Self-determination and personal freedom: Self-love enables us to determine our own direction in life and to live authentically. We do not allow ourselves to be limited by the expectations of others or social norms. Instead, we follow our inner voice and shape our lives according to our own desires and needs.

12. Self-Care and Self-Nourishing Practices: Self-love involves the conscious care and nourishment of our body, mind, and soul. We regularly set aside time for self-care practices such as meditation, yoga, being close to nature, creative activities or reading inspirational books. These practices give us energy, strengthen our self-love, and promote our holistic healing.

The power of self-love is limitless. By reminding ourselves daily to love and accept ourselves unconditionally, we can anchor ourselves in our innermost being and express our true essence. Self-love is a lifelong process that encourages us to dive deeper and deeper into our own love and reach our full potential.

In this chapter we have highlighted the many aspects of self-love. I encourage you to continue to grow in your own self-love and integrate this healing power into your daily life. By strengthening your self-love, you will not only experience your own wholeness and healing, but also give other people a shining example of how they themselves can cultivate love and healing in their lives.

Be patient and compassionate with yourself on this path of self-love. They deserve to love themselves and live a full, authentic life. Discover the infinite power of self-love and let it transform your world.

Chapter 16: Sleep and Recovery: The Underrated Healer

In the previous chapters, we covered in detail the various aspects of self-healing, from diet and exercise to mental health and social relationships. In this chapter, we focus on two often underestimated but crucial elements of the healing process: sleep and recovery.

The Science of Sleep

Sleep is not simply a "time out" for the body and mind; it is an active period in which a number of important regeneration and repair processes take place. During sleep, the body goes through different sleep cycles, including REM (rapid eye movement) and non-REM phases, each of which has specific functions for physical and mental health.

Immune system

One of the most important systems that is activated during sleep is the immune system. Studies have shown that chronic lack of sleep can lead to a weakening of the immune system, increasing susceptibility to infections and diseases.

Mental health

Mental health also benefits enormously from good sleep. Lack of sleep can lead to a number of mental health problems, including depression, anxiety, and stress. During sleep, neurotransmitters are rebalanced, and the brain performs a kind of "self-purification" that is crucial for emotional and cognitive function.

Physical regeneration

Sleep is also the time when the body repairs itself. Cells are renewed, tissues are repaired and muscles are built. This is especially important for people recovering from injury or surgery.

Techniques for better sleep

Sleep hygiene

Sleep hygiene refers to a set of habits and practices that promote healthy sleep. These include a constant sleep time, a comfortable sleeping environment and the absence of electronic devices before bedtime.

Relaxation

Methods such as meditation, progressive muscle relaxation, or breathing exercises can help calm the mind and prepare the body for sleep.

Nutrition and sleep

Certain foods can promote or disrupt sleep. A light dinner that's high in magnesium and low in caffeine and sugar can improve sleep.

The importance of recovery

In addition to sleep, recovery while awake is also crucial for self-healing. Recovery is important not only physically, but also psychologically.

Active and passive recreation

Active recreation refers to activities that require physical or mental effort, but are still perceived as refreshing and renewing. Passive recovery, on the other hand, involves activities that require little to no effort, such as taking a nap or reading a book.

The role of nature

As mentioned in a previous chapter, nature has a healing effect. Spending time in nature can be seen as a form of recreation that revitalizes both the body and mind.

Summary and conclusions

Sleep and recovery are essential components of the self-healing process. They provide an opportunity for the body and mind to regenerate and repair, which is crucial for maintaining health and well-being. By implementing techniques for better sleep and conscious recovery, we can actively support and promote the healing process.

In this chapter, we've explored the science behind sleep and recovery, as well as practical techniques to improve both. Incorporating these principles into your everyday life is another step in your journey to self-healing.

Remember that self-healing is an ongoing process that requires dedication and patience. Sleep and recovery are not "luxury goods", but necessary components of this process. By giving them the attention they deserve, you're taking another important step in your journey to holistic health and well-being.

Chapter 17: The Role of Creativity and Expression in Self-Healing

Creativity is often seen as a luxury or the talent of a few people. In truth, however, it is a universal human need and a powerful resource for self-healing. In this chapter, we will explore the many ways in which creative expressions such as painting, writing, dancing, and music can have therapeutic effects. We will also provide practical guidance on how to use your own creativity as part of your healing process.

Why creativity is important

Creativity is not just an expression of talent or ability; it is also a means of self-discovery, processing emotions and promoting psychological well-being. Creative activities can be seen as a form of "inner work" that allows us to better understand ourselves and our inner worlds.

Creativity and the brain

Neuroscience studies have shown that creative activities such as painting or making music activate areas of the brain associated with emotions, memory and self-awareness. This activation can lead to the release of neurotransmitters such as dopamine, which promote feelings of well-being and relaxation.

Creativity and Emotional Intelligence

Creative expressions provide a safe platform to explore and process emotions. Whether it's writing a diary, painting a picture, or composing a song, the creative process allows us to channel our feelings in a constructive way.

Creative forms of therapy

There are a number of recognized forms of therapy that use creativity as a means of healing. These include art therapy, music therapy, dance therapy, and writing therapy. These forms of therapy are often used in clinical settings, but can also be practiced in a personal setting.

Art therapy

In art therapy, participants use visual media such as painting, drawing, or sculpture to express their thoughts and feelings. The creative process itself and the subsequent interpretation of the artworks can offer deep insights into emotional and psychological states.

Music therapy

Music therapy uses music to promote physical and emotional healing. This can be done by listening to music, playing instruments, or even writing songs. Music has the ability to penetrate deep into our emotions and can serve as a powerful tool for mood regulation.

Dance Therapy

Dance therapy combines movement and music to improve physical and emotional health. Through dance, participants can express their emotions while promoting their physical fitness.

Writing Therapy

Writing therapy, often referred to as "therapeutic writing," is a method in which writing is used as a tool for exploring and processing emotions. This can be in the form of diary writing, poetry or even fictional writing.

Practical applications

Creativity in everyday life

You don't have to be a professional artist or musician to reap the benefits of creativity. Simple activities like drawing doodles, writing poetry, or dancing in your living room can have therapeutic effects.

Creative exercises

1. **Free Writing**: Take 15 minutes to write non-stop. Ignore grammar and spelling and let your thoughts flow freely.
2. **Paint by Feeling**: Choose colors that reflect your current mood and let your brush dance on the canvas.
3. **Spontaneous Dance**: Put on your favorite music and let your body move freely as it wants.

Inference

Creativity is an often overlooked but powerful ally on the path of self-healing. By incorporating creative practices into your healing process, you can not only improve your emotional and mental health, but also develop a deeper understanding of yourself. Whether you choose art, music, dance, or writing, the key is to find a creative expression that has meaning to you personally and allows you to express yourself authentically.

In this chapter, we explored the scientific and therapeutic basis of creativity as a tool for self-healing. We've also featured practical exercises and tips that you can incorporate into your own healing process. As with all other aspects of self-healing, the most important step you can take is the first. So, take that pen, brush, or dance shoes and start your own creative journey to healing.

Chapter 18: Technology and Self-Healing: Friend or Foe?

In this day and age, technology is ubiquitous. It has the potential to improve our lives in many ways, but it also comes with challenges, especially when it comes to our health and well-being. In this chapter, we will explore the dual role of technology in the context of self-healing: how can it support us, and how can it harm us? And above all, how can we consciously use them to promote our self-healing powers?

Technology as a support for self-healing

Health Apps

There are a variety of health apps out there, ranging from physical activity monitoring to meditation. These apps can help us better track and achieve our health goals. They can also serve as a reminder to incorporate healthy habits into our daily lives.

Telemedicine

Telemedicine allows us to receive medical advice and treatment remotely. This is especially useful for people who live in remote areas or have difficulty seeing a doctor in person. Telemedicine can also serve as a complementary resource for self-healing by providing quick access to expertise.

Wearables

Wearable devices like smartwatches can collect a wealth of health data, from heart rate to sleep patterns. This data can give us valuable insights into our state of health and serve as a basis for targeted self-healing measures.

Technology as a challenge for self-healing

Technology-induced stress

The constant availability and the flood of information can lead to stress and excessive demands. This can have a negative impact on our mental health and hinder the self-healing process.

Screen Time and Physical Health

Excessive screen time is associated with a number of health problems, including eye strain, poor posture, and lack of exercise. These factors can impair the body's self-healing powers.

Social Media and Mental Health

Although social media provides an opportunity to connect with others, it can also lead to feelings of isolation and comparison, which negatively impact mental health.

Strategies for the conscious use of technology

Digital Detox

A "digital detox" can be an effective way to minimize the negative effects of technology. This can be as simple as setting specific times to stay away from all digital devices.

Setting boundaries

Setting boundaries on the use of technology can help reduce technology-induced stress. This can be achieved by using app limits or special "Screen Time" settings on your devices.

Choosing the right tools

Not all technologies are created equal. It's important to consciously choose which technologies and apps best fit your self-healing goals. Read reviews, do your research, and experiment to find out which tools are most effective for you.

Inference

Technology is a double-edged sword in the context of self-healing. While it has the potential to support us in a variety of ways, it also comes with challenges and risks. The key lies in conscious use: by being aware of the pros and cons and implementing proactive strategies to minimize the risks, we can reap the benefits of technology without compromising our health.

In this chapter, we explored the different aspects of technology in the context of self-healing. We looked at both the positive and negative effects and presented strategies on how to consciously use technology to promote self-healing. As with all other aspects of self-healing, it's important that you use technology in a way that suits your individual needs and circumstances. It's another tool in your self-healing arsenal – use it wisely.

Chapter 19: The importance of self-forgiveness in the healing process

Self-criticism, guilt and self-reproach can be significant obstacles on the way to self-healing. These mental and emotional blockages can not only slow down the healing process, but also cause further health problems. In this chapter, we will examine the practice of self-forgiveness as a crucial factor in the healing process. We will present techniques and strategies that can help you forgive yourself and thus pave the way for effective self-healing.

Why is self-forgiveness important?

Psychological aspects

Self-forgiveness can be seen as an act of self-love and self-compassion. Psychological studies have shown that people who can forgive themselves are less prone to depression, anxiety and stress. These factors can significantly affect the self-healing process.

Physiological aspects

The ability to self-forgive can even have physiological effects. Stress and negative emotions can weaken the immune system and promote inflammation in the body. So, by reducing these negative emotions through self-forgiveness, you can also improve your physical health.

Obstacles on the way to self-forgiveness

Guilt and shame

Guilt and shame are often the biggest obstacles on the road to self-forgiveness. These emotions can be deep-rooted and require a conscious effort to overcome them.

Fear of weakness

Many people see self-forgiveness as a sign of weakness. They believe that they need to punish themselves in order to learn from their mistakes. However, this attitude can be counterproductive and hinder the healing process.

Cultural and societal norms

In some cultures and societies, self-criticism is encouraged and seen as a virtue. This can make it difficult to see the value of self-forgiveness and put it into practice.

Techniques to promote self-forgiveness

Mindfulness meditation

Mindfulness meditation can help you observe your thoughts and feelings without judgment. This can be the first step to self-forgiveness, as it allows you to recognize and let go of your self-criticism.

Journaling

Writing a journal can be a powerful tool for self-reflection. By writing down your thoughts and feelings, you can take a step back and better understand why you judge yourself so harshly.

Affirmations

Positive affirmations can help you change your thought patterns. By regularly repeating positive phrases, you can improve your self-awareness and pave the way for self-forgiveness.

Therapy and counseling

Sometimes the obstacles to self-forgiveness can be so great that professional help is required. Therapists can offer specific techniques and exercises tailored to your individual needs.

Case studies

Case study 1: Anna and self-forgiveness after a failed relationship

Anna could not forgive herself after their long-term relationship failed. She blamed herself for everything and suffered from severe depression. Through therapy and the practice of mindfulness meditation, she learned to forgive herself. This led not only to an improvement in their mental health, but also to a strengthening of their immune system.

Case Study 2: Mark and Self-Forgiveness in the Context of a Chronic Illness

Markus, who suffered from a chronic illness, blamed himself for believing that he had not done enough for his health. Through journaling and positive affirmations, he was able to let go of these self-destructive thoughts. This had a positive impact on his overall health and promoted his self-healing powers.

Inference

Self-forgiveness is not just a psychological exercise, but an integral part of the self-healing process. It affects both our mental and physical health and can pave the way for effective and sustainable self-healing. Through various techniques such as mindfulness meditation, journaling, positive affirmations and professional therapy, we can learn to forgive ourselves and thus promote our well-being on all levels.

In this chapter, we have explored in detail the importance of self-forgiveness in the healing process. We have identified obstacles that can prevent us from forgiving ourselves and presented techniques that can support us on this path. The ability to self-forgive is a valuable tool in your arsenal for self-healing. It's never too late to incorporate this practice into your life and enjoy the many benefits it offers.

Chapter 20: The Journey of Self-Healing: Case Studies and Success Stories

Now that we've worked our way through the various aspects of self-healing, from the importance of nutrition to the power of self-forgiveness, it's time to put the theory into practice. In this concluding chapter, we present case studies and personal stories of people who have successfully gone through the process of self-healing. These inspiring stories serve as examples of what's possible and offer hands-on insights into the challenges and triumphs that can occur on this journey.

Case Study 1: Lisa – The Power of Nutrition

Lisa, a 42-year-old woman, suffered from type 2 diabetes and was overweight. She had tried various medications, but the side effects were bothering her. Eventually, she decided to radically change her lifestyle. She began to eat healthily by eliminating industrially processed foods and sugar from her diet. After six months, she found that her blood sugar levels had normalized and she had lost weight. Her doctors were amazed and adjusted her medication accordingly. Lisa is a living example of how powerful proper nutrition can be.

Case Study 2: Ahmed – Mindfulness and Stress Management

Ahmed, a 35-year-old software developer, suffered from chronic stress and burnout. He hardly found time for himself and constantly felt exhausted. After reading several articles about the benefits of mindfulness, he decided to give it a try. He began to meditate daily and take mindful walks. Within a few weeks, he noticed a significant improvement in his stress levels and overall quality of life. Ahmed's story shows how mindfulness and stress management can go hand in hand to promote self-healing.

Case Study 3: Elena – The Healing Power of Nature

Elena, a 50-year-old teacher, suffered from depression and anxiety. She had tried different medications and therapies, but nothing seemed to help. Then she discovered the healing power of nature. She began to regularly hike in nature and spend time outdoors. She noticed that her mood improved and her anxiety symptoms subsided. Elena is proof that nature can be a powerful ally on the path of self-healing.

Case Study 4: Tom – The Power of Positive Relationships

Tom, a 60-year-old retiree, felt lonely and isolated after the death of his wife. He withdrew from friends and family and fell into depression. It wasn't until he joined a community group and began socializing that his condition changed. The positive relationships he built helped him come out of his isolation and rediscover his zest for life. Tom's story shows how important positive relationships can be for mental and physical health.

Case Study 5: Sophie – Technology as a Friend

Sophie, a 28-year-old marketing manager, suffered from chronic back pain. She had already tried different therapeutic approaches, but nothing seemed to work. Then she discovered an app for physiotherapy exercises and started using it regularly. The app helped her to perform the exercises correctly and motivated her to keep at it. Within a few months, her back pain was significantly better. Sophie shows that technology, when used correctly, can be a powerful tool for self-healing.

Common findings and conclusions

The stories of these people show that self-healing is a multi-layered process that includes physical, mental and emotional aspects. They also show that there is no one-size-fits-all solution; what works for one person doesn't necessarily work for another. The key is to try different approaches and see what works best for you.

It is also important to emphasize that self-healing is an ongoing process. It's not a "once-and-done" thing, but requires continuous effort and adaptation. But as these stories show, it's a journey worth it. Every little step you take brings you closer to a life of health and well-being.

Chapter 21: Conclusion: The Continuous Pursuit of Health and Well-Being

Congratulations! You have now reached the conclusion of this guide to self-healing. We hope that you have gained valuable insights and inspiration for your own path to health and well-being.

In this concluding chapter, we would like to give you some important thoughts and recommendations to help you maintain and deepen your pursuit of health and well-being.

1. Continuity and commitment: Self-healing is an ongoing process that requires your attention and dedication. Take time for yourself to take care of your health and work on your goals. Stay consistent in your efforts and don't be discouraged by setbacks.

2. Reflection and adaptation: Take time regularly to reflect on your progress and review your strategies. Ask yourself: What worked well? What could be improved? Adapt your approach and experiment with new approaches to meet your individual needs.

3. Network and Support: Surround yourself with a supportive community. Share your experiences, challenges and successes with others. Together you can motivate and inspire each other. Look for support groups, online forums, or health events to connect with like-minded people.

4. Self-care: Don't forget to take good care of yourself. Take regular breaks to relax and recharge. Practice mindfulness, meditation, or other techniques to calm your mind and reduce stress. Listen to your body's needs and give yourself enough sleep, a healthy diet and physical exercise.

5. Evolution: The pursuit of health and well-being never stops. Stay open to new insights and opportunities for further education. Read books, attend seminars, or look for experts to help you expand your knowledge and skills.

Finally, we would like to thank you again for your time and interest in this self-healing guide. Remember that the power to self-heal lies within you. Be confident in your abilities and implement the strategies and techniques presented in this book.

May this guide accompany you on your journey to health and well-being and help you live a full and healthy life. We wish you all the best!

In the appendix of this guide, you will find a collection of helpful resources and exercises that can help you on your journey to self-healing. These additional materials can help you deepen your knowledge, improve your skills, and further promote your health and well-being. Let's take a look at some of the resources and exercises you'll find here:

1. Recommended Books: A list of books on self-healing, health, nutrition, exercise, mental health, and other related topics. These books provide in-depth information, inspiring stories, and practical guidance to support your self-healing journey.

2. Online Resources: A selection of websites, blogs, podcasts, and videos dedicated to self-healing, health, and wellbeing. Here you will find more information, expert interviews, guides and advice that can accompany you on your way.

3. Mindfulness Exercises: A collection of mindfulness exercises to help you be aware of the moment, calm your mind, and reduce stress. From breathing exercises to meditation to mindful eating, here are various techniques to help you be present in the here and now.

4. Physical exercises: A set of physical exercises that will help you strengthen your body, improve flexibility and increase your well-being. From yoga poses to stretching exercises to full-body workouts , there are several options you can choose from.

5. Journaling: Keeping a journal can help you reflect on your thoughts and feelings, record your goals, and record your progress. Here are guides for various journaling techniques that can help you gain clarity and document your self-healing journey.

6. Support Groups and Communities: A list of local and online support groups and communities where you can connect with like-minded people, get advice, and motivate each other. Sharing your experiences and challenges with others can be a valuable support on your journey.

These resources and exercises are intended to complement the information and strategies presented in this book. Use them as tools to expand your knowledge, deepen your practice, and develop your self-healing skills.

We hope this appendix will provide you with helpful support and help you take your health and well-being to new heights. Remember that self-healing is a lifelong journey characterized by patience, dedication, and a willingness to constantly evolve. There is no end point, only new opportunities for improvement and growth. Stay curious, stay engaged, and most importantly, be gentle with yourself along the way.

We wish you continued success and satisfaction on your journey to self-healing, health and well-being. May each day bring you new insights and joys.

Best wishes!

Epilogue

You've reached the end of this comprehensive guide, and we hope your journey through the pages of Heal Yourself: A Guide to Self-Healing has been both enlightening and empowering. When you close this book, a new chapter opens in your life – one in which you have the tools and knowledge to actively shape your health and well-being.

The goal of this book was to inspire you to recognize and harness the incredible power of self-healing. We've covered a variety of topics, from the physiology of the body and the importance of a balanced diet to the subtle yet powerful forces of the mind and spirit. Each chapter should be seen as a step towards a holistic understanding of your own health.

It is important to emphasize that the journey of self-healing is an ongoing one. Health, as mentioned several times in the book, is not a goal, but a process. It is a dynamic balance that requires constant attention and care. With the tools and strategies presented in this book, you'll be better prepared to be aware and proactive about this process.

Another important aspect is the individuality of the healing process. What works for one person doesn't necessarily work for another. Therefore, it is crucial that you adapt the methods and techniques presented in this book to your own needs and life circumstances. Self-healing is a very personal journey shaped by your own intuition, experiences, and commitment.

We hope that the insights and techniques you have gained from this book will guide you on your journey to a healthier, more fulfilling life. May the journey of self-healing that you have now embarked on lead you to new heights of well-being and self-knowledge.

Thank you for your time and dedication. We wish you all the best for the future.

Yours sincerely,

Printed in Great Britain
by Amazon

27590618R10037